THE TESTOSTERONE
ADVANTAGE
COOKBOOK

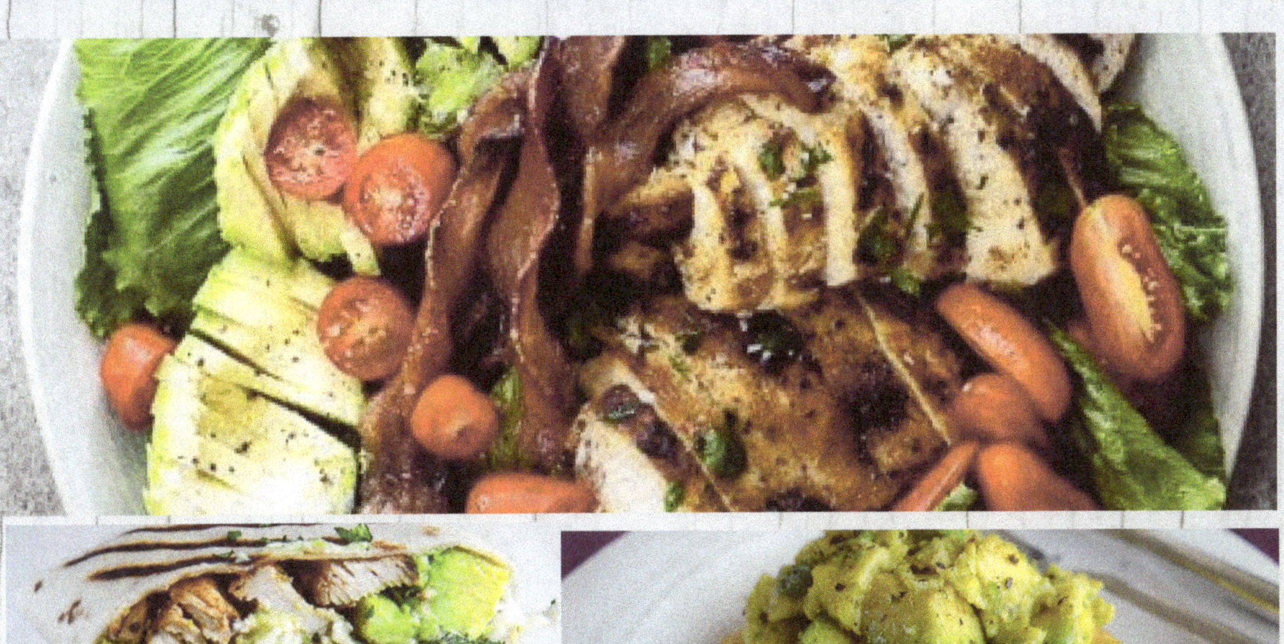

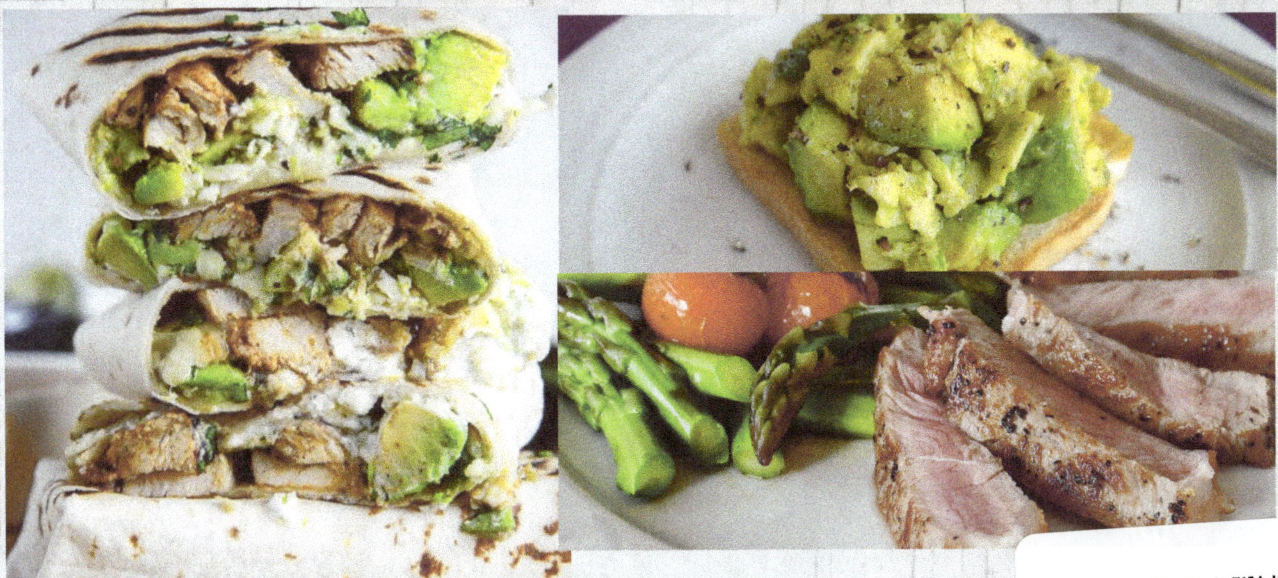

ANTHONY ALEXIS

TABLE OF CONTENTS

1 INTRODUCTION

TESTOSTERONE BOOSTING FOODS 7

2 BREAKFAST

10 DAYS TESTOSTERONE BOOSTING 13
BREAKFAST RECIPES.
BREAKFAST MENU 27

3 LUNCH

10 DAYS TESTOSTERONE BOOSTING 32
LUNCH RECIPES.
LUNCH MENU 45

4 DINNER

10 DAYS TESTOSTERONE BOOSTING 48
DINNER RECIPES.
DINNER MENU 59

TABLE OF CONTENTS

5 TESTOSTERONE BOOSTING SNACKS AND DRINKS 65

6 OVERCOMING NUTRITION CHALLENGES 66

7 SUSTAINING THE TESTOSTERONE ADVANTAGE: LONG TERM 70

INTRODUCTION

As men, we often take our bodily functions for granted. We rarely stop to consider the intricate interplay of hormones and neurotransmitters that orchestrate our health, performance, and overall well-being. Testosterone, the primary male sex hormone, plays a pivotal role in shaping our physical and mental landscapes.

I've always been fascinated by the concept of testosterone. It's the hormone that fuels our masculine identity, the driving force behind our physical development, and the silent regulator of our emotions and motivations. As a man who has experienced the fluctuations of testosterone levels throughout my life, I've come to appreciate the profound impact this hormone has on my overall health and performance.

During my teenage years, testosterone was the catalyst for my growth spurts, the deepening of my voice, and the surge in energy that fueled my athletic pursuits. It was the hormone that transformed me from a lanky boy into a young man, instilling in me a sense of confidence and self-assurance.

As I transitioned into adulthood, testosterone's influence evolved from the physical realm to the mental and emotional spheres. It became the quiet force that kept me motivated, focused, and resilient in the face of challenges. It was the energy that propelled me through long workdays and demanding academic pursuits. It was the spark that ignited my passions and fueled my determination to succeed.

However, testosterone's impact is not limited to physical and mental performance; it extends to our overall health and well-being as well. Testosterone plays a crucial role in maintaining muscle mass, bone density, and red blood cell production. It contributes to a healthy immune system and supports the production of sperm.

While testosterone is often associated with aggression and virility, it also plays a role in regulating mood, libido, and cognitive function. When testosterone levels are optimal, we experience a sense of well-being, confidence, and emotional stability.

We're more likely to feel energized, motivated, and capable of taking on the world.

However, when testosterone levels dip, we may experience a range of negative symptoms. Fatigue, mood swings, irritability, and a decline in libido are common manifestations of low testosterone. We may find it harder to concentrate, make decisions, and maintain our energy levels.

Maintaining optimal testosterone levels is essential for both men's physical and mental health. It's a critical component of overall well-being, contributing to our ability to thrive in all aspects of life. By understanding the profound impact of testosterone, we can take steps to optimize our hormone balance and reap the benefits of a healthy, balanced life.

The Role of Diet in Testosterone Production.

As a man who has always been health-conscious, I've always been intrigued by the role that nutrition plays in optimizing testosterone levels. Over the years, I've experimented with various dietary approaches, from high-protein diets to intermittent fasting, observing how my body responds and how it affects my overall well-being.

One of the most significant insights I've gained is the profound impact that diet has on testosterone production. Certain nutrients, such as zinc, magnesium, and vitamin D, play crucial roles in regulating testosterone levels. Consuming adequate amounts of these nutrients through a balanced and varied diet can help maintain optimal hormone balance.

Zinc, a mineral found in meats, seafood, nuts, and legumes, is essential for testosterone synthesis and metabolism. It also supports sperm production and male reproductive health. Magnesium, another essential mineral, is involved in various bodily processes, including testosterone production and regulation. It also contributes to muscle function, energy production, and stress management. Vitamin D, often referred to as the "sunshine vitamin," is also critical for testosterone production and overall health. Our bodies can produce vitamin D when exposed to sunlight, but many people don't get enough sun exposure, making dietary sources essential.

Vitamin D-rich foods include fatty fish, eggs, and fortified dairy products.

In addition to these essential nutrients, overall dietary patterns can also influence testosterone levels. A diet rich in fruits, vegetables, whole grains, and lean proteins provides the body with the nutrients it needs to function optimally, supporting testosterone production and overall health.

On the other hand, diets high in processed foods, sugary drinks, and excessive saturated and unhealthy fats can negatively impact testosterone levels. These foods can contribute to inflammation, insulin resistance, and overall metabolic dysfunction, all of which can interfere with testosterone production.

My personal experience has shown that making conscious dietary choices can significantly impact my testosterone levels and overall well-being. When I focus on consuming nutrient-rich foods and limiting processed options, I notice an increase in energy levels, improved mood, and enhanced cognitive function. These changes have translated into better performance in both physical and mental aspects of my life.

TESTOSTERONE BOOSTING FOODS

As a man who has always been passionate about health and fitness, I've come to appreciate the profound impact that nutrition plays in optimizing testosterone levels. Testosterone, the primary male sex hormone, is crucial for maintaining muscle mass, bone density, red blood cell production, and overall well-being. It also contributes to a healthy immune system, supports sperm production, and regulates mood, libido, and cognitive function.

I will list few classes foods that effectively boosts the testosterone:

1. Zinc

Zinc is an essential mineral that plays a critical role in testosterone synthesis and metabolism. It's also involved in sperm production and male reproductive health. Adequate zinc intake is crucial for maintaining optimal testosterone levels.

Food Sources of Zinc:

Oysters: Oysters are the richest dietary source of zinc, providing over 700% of the daily recommended intake (RDI) in a single serving.
Beef: Beef is another excellent source of zinc, providing about 40% of the RDI per serving.
Pumpkin Seeds: Pumpkin seeds are a plant-based source of zinc, providing about 20% of the RDI per serving.
Dark Chocolate: Dark chocolate contains zinc in addition to other beneficial nutrients like magnesium and antioxidants.

2. Magnesium

Magnesium is another essential mineral that plays a vital role in testosterone production and regulation.

It's also involved in muscle function, energy production, and stress management. Adequate magnesium intake is essential for maintaining optimal testosterone levels.

Food Sources of Magnesium:

Leafy Green Vegetables: Leafy green vegetables like spinach, kale, and collard greens are excellent sources of magnesium.

Nuts and Seeds: Nuts and seeds like almonds, cashews, and sunflower seeds are rich in magnesium.

Whole Grains: Whole grains like brown rice, quinoa, and oats provide magnesium along with other essential nutrients.

Vitamin D

Vitamin D, often referred to as the "sunshine vitamin," is also crucial for testosterone production and overall health. It's involved in calcium absorption, bone health, and immune function. Adequate vitamin D intake is essential for maintaining optimal testosterone levels.

Food Sources of Vitamin D:

Fatty Fish: Fatty fish like salmon, sardines, and mackerel are excellent sources of vitamin D.
Egg Yolks: Egg yolks contain vitamin D, along with other nutrients like protein and choline.
Fortified Foods: Many foods, such as milk, cereal, and orange juice, are fortified with vitamin D.

Incorporating Testosterone-Boosting Foods into Your Diet
By incorporating foods rich in zinc, magnesium, and vitamin D into your diet, you can support optimal testosterone production and overall health. Here are some tips for incorporating these nutrient-rich foods into your meals:

Start your day with a zinc-rich breakfast: Enjoy an omelet with zinc-rich oysters or a bowl of oatmeal topped with zinc-rich pumpkin seeds.

Incorporate magnesium-rich vegetables into your meals: Include leafy green vegetables like spinach and kale in your salads, stir-fries, and soups.

Snack on magnesium-rich nuts and seeds:.Keep a handful of nuts and seeds on hand for a healthy and satisfying snack.

Include fatty fish in your diet: Enjoy salmon, sardines, or mackerel for a delicious and nutritious meal.

Consume egg yolks: Include egg yolks in your omelets, scrambled eggs, or as a topping for salads and sandwiches.

Choose fortified foods:.Opt for fortified milk, cereal, and orange juice to boost your vitamin D intake.

Consistency is key. By making conscious dietary choices and incorporating these nutrient-rich foods into your daily routine, you can support optimal testosterone levels and experience a range of health benefits.

Protein-Rich Foods for Muscle Growth and Testosterone Production.

The Role of Protein in Muscle Growth and Testosterone Production.

As an avid fitness enthusiast, I've always been fascinated by the complex interplay between nutrition, exercise, and hormone production. Protein, in particular, plays a pivotal role in muscle growth and repair, and it also has a significant impact on testosterone levels, the primary male sex hormone.
Protein's Impact on Muscle Growth.
Protein is the building block of muscle tissue. When we engage in resistance training, we create microscopic tears in our muscles. These tears are then repaired through a process called muscle protein synthesis (MPS), which requires ample amounts of protein.

Consuming adequate protein after resistance training stimulates MPS, leading to muscle growth and repair. The amount of protein needed varies depending on individual factors such as age, activity level, and training goals. However, a general guideline is to consume around 0.8 grams of protein per kilogram of body weight per day.

Protein's Impact on Testosterone Production.

Protein also plays a role in testosterone production. Amino acids, the building blocks of protein, are involved in the synthesis of testosterone. Studies have shown that higher protein intake can lead to increased testosterone levels.

In addition to its direct impact on testosterone production, protein also contributes to overall health and well-being. It supports a healthy immune system, strengthens bones and connective tissues, and aids in energy production.

Incorporating Protein-Rich Foods into Your Diet

There are many excellent sources of protein that can be easily incorporated into a healthy diet. Here are a few examples:

Lean meats: Chicken, turkey, fish, and lean cuts of beef are all excellent sources of protein.

Eggs: Eggs are a versatile and nutrient-rich source of protein.

Dairy products: Milk, yogurt, and cheese provide protein along with calcium and other essential nutrients.

Plant-based sources: Beans, lentils, tofu, and tempeh are all excellent sources of plant-based protein.

Personal Experience

As a personal trainer, I've seen firsthand the impact that protein intake has o has on my clients' muscle growth and overall fitness goals. By incorporating protein-rich foods into their diets, they've experienced increased muscle mass, improved strength, and enhanced energy levels.

I've also noticed the positive impact of protein intake on my own fitness journey. When I prioritize protein-rich foods, I feel more energized, focused, and able to perform at my best during workouts.

Testosterone-Boosting Fruits and Vegetables
Harnessing the Power of Plant-Based Testosterone Boosters

As a man committed to maintaining optimal health, I've always been intrigued by the role that nutrition plays in optimizing hormone balance, particularly testosterone. While protein, zinc, magnesium, and vitamin D are often at the forefront of testosterone-boosting discussions, the power of fruits and vegetables should not be overlooked.

Citrus Fruits
Citrus fruits, such as oranges, grapefruits, and lemons, are rich in vitamin C, a powerful antioxidant that supports testosterone production and overall immune function. Studies have shown that vitamin C supplementation can increase testosterone levels in individuals with low vitamin C status.

Berries
Berries, including strawberries, blueberries, and raspberries, are packed with antioxidants and anti-inflammatory compounds that can positively impact testosterone levels. Studies have shown that berry consumption can reduce oxidative stress, a factor that can contribute to low testosterone levels.

Pomegranate
Pomegranate, a unique and flavorful fruit, has been shown to significantly boost testosterone levels. Studies have demonstrated that pomegranate consumption can increase testosterone by up to 24% in men with low testosterone levels.

Watermelon

Watermelon, a refreshing and hydrating fruit, contains lycopene, an antioxidant that may support testosterone production. Lycopene has also been shown to improve sperm quality and motility.

Grapes

Grapes, particularly red grapes, contain resveratrol, a compound that has shown promise in boosting testosterone levels. Resveratrol has anti-inflammatory properties and may also improve blood flow.

Incorporating Testosterone-Boosting Fruits and Vegetables into Your Diet.

Adding a variety of fruits and vegetables to your diet is not only beneficial for testosterone production but also for overall health and well-being. Here are some tips for incorporating these nutrient-rich foods into your daily routine:

Start your day with a fruit-infused breakfast: Enjoy a smoothie packed with berries, pomegranate seeds, or sliced citrus fruits.

Incorporate salads into your meals: Add colorful fruits like strawberries, blueberries, or grapes to your salads for a burst of flavor and nutrients.

Make fruit your go-to snack: Instead of reaching for processed snacks, grab a handful of berries, slices of watermelon, or a fresh orange.

Include vegetables in your dinner: Enjoy grilled or roasted vegetables as a side dish or incorporate them into stir-fries and soups.

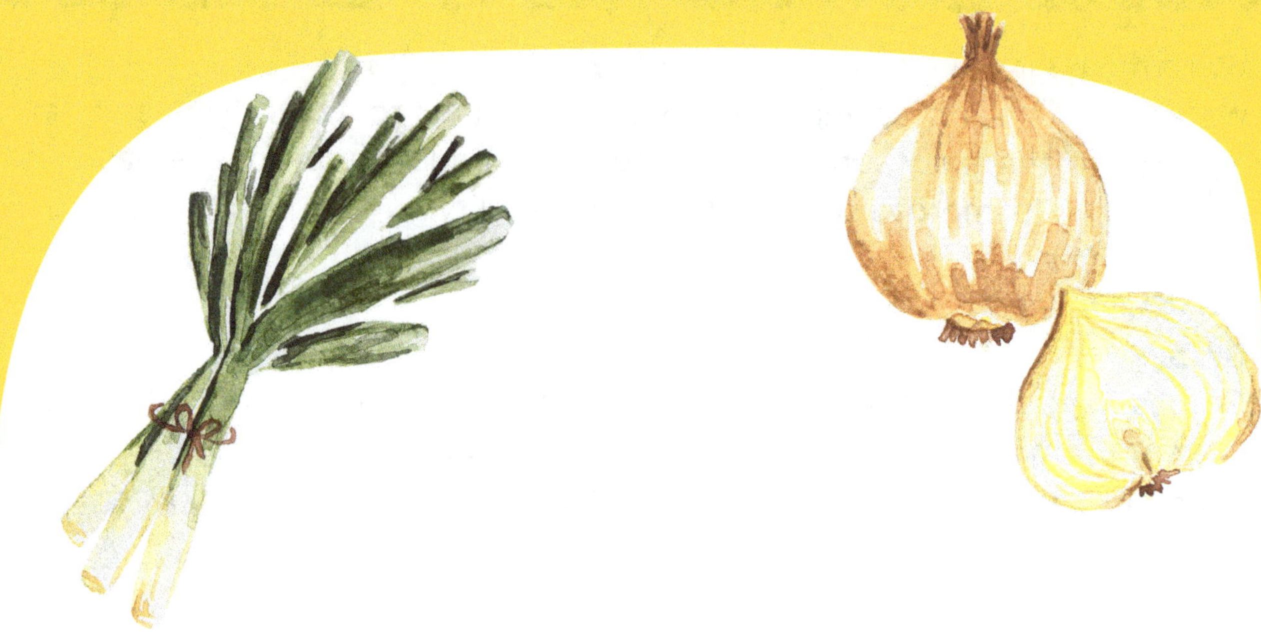

TESTOSTERONE-BOOSTING BREAKFAST RECIPES

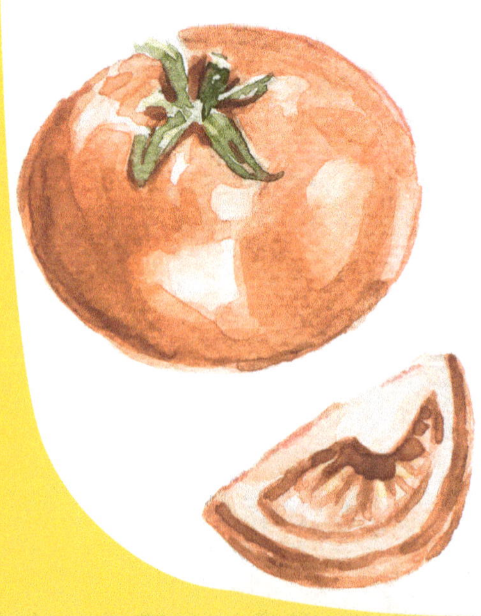

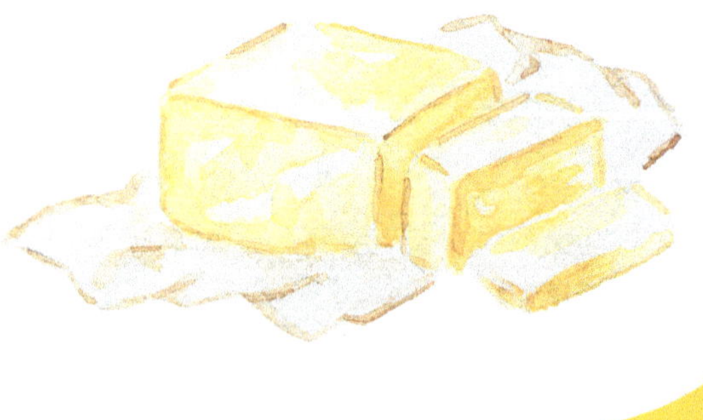

HIGH-PROTEIN OMELET WITH TESTOSTERONE-ENHANCING INGREDIENTS

INGREDIENTS

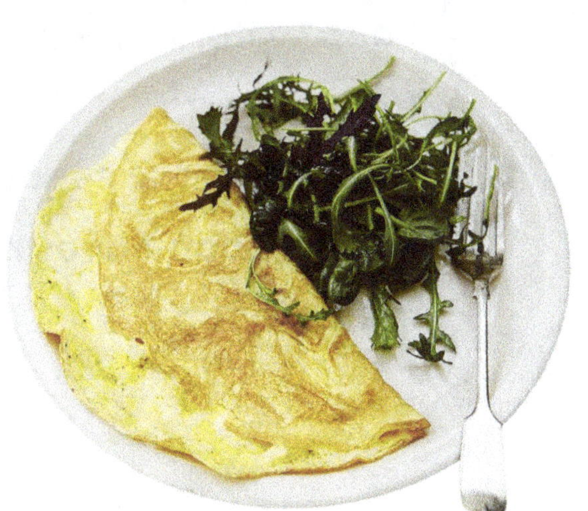

- **2 eggs**
- **1 tablespoon olive oil**
- **1/4 cup chopped spinach**
- **1/4 cup shredded mushrooms**
- **1/4 cup chopped bell peppers**
- **1/4 cup cooked turkey sausage**
- **1 tablespoon grated Parmesan cheese**

INSTRUCTIONS

1. Whisk eggs together in a bowl.
2. Heat olive oil in a skillet over medium heat.
3. Add spinach, mushrooms, and bell peppers to the skillet and cook until softened.
4. Add cooked turkey sausage to the skillet and crumble with a spatula.
5. Pour whisked eggs into the skillet and cook until the bottom is set.
6. Sprinkle Parmesan cheese over the omelet and fold in half.
7. Serve immediately.

TESTOSTERONE-ENHANCING OATMEAL BOWL

INGREDIENTS

- 1/2 cup rolled oats
- 1 cup water or milk
- 1/4 cup berries
- 1/4 cup nuts or seeds
- 1 tablespoon honey or maple syrup

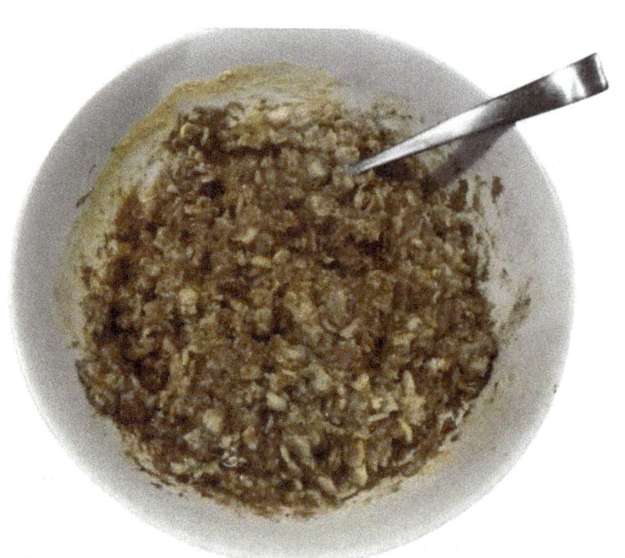

INSTRUCTIONS

1. In a small saucepan, bring water or milk to a boil over medium heat.
2. Add rolled oats to the saucepan and reduce heat to low.
3. Simmer for 5-7 minutes, or until oats are cooked through.
4. Stir in berries, nuts or seeds, and honey or maple syrup.
5. Enjoy immediately.

TESTOSTERONE-ENHANCING SMOOTHIE

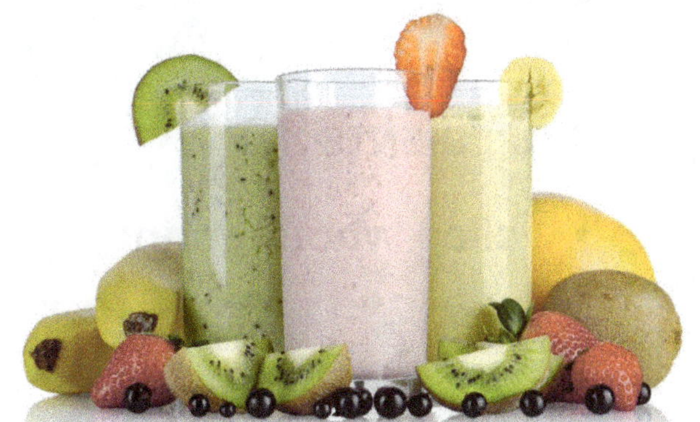

INGREDIENTS

- 1 cup spinach
- 1 banana
- 1/2 cup berries
- 1 scoop protein powder
- 1 cup milk or yogurt

INSTRUCTIONS

1. Combine all ingredients in a blender and blend until smooth.
2. Enjoy

TESTOSTERONE-ENHANCING AVOCADO TOAST

INGREDIENTS

- 1 slice whole-grain toast
- 1/2 avocado, mashed
- 1 tablespoon pomegranate seeds
- 1 tablespoon hemp seeds

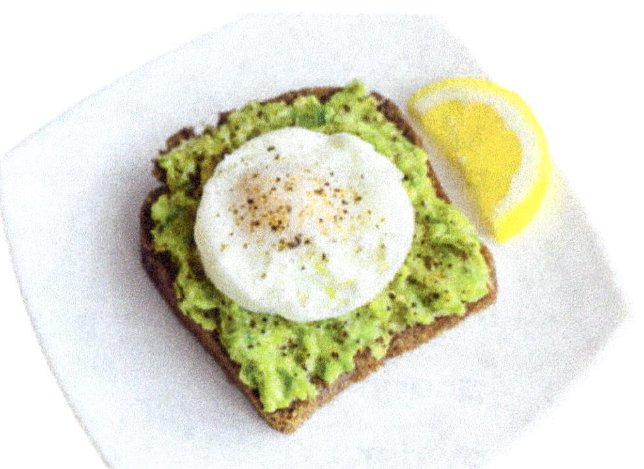

INSTRUCTIONS

1. Toast bread to your liking.
2. Spread mashed avocado on toast.
3. Top with pomegranate seeds and hemp seeds.
4. Enjoy immediately.

TESTOSTERONE-ENHANCING GREEK YOGURT PARFAIT

INGREDIENTS

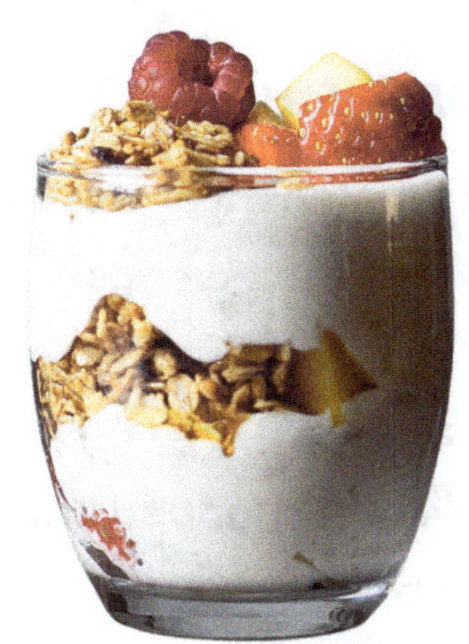

- **1 cup plain Greek yogurt**
- **1/4 cup berries**
- **1/4 cup granola**

INSTRUCTIONS

1. Layer Greek yogurt, berries, and granola in a glass or parfait cup.
2. Enjoy immediately.

TESTOSTERONE-ENHANCING BREAKFAST BURRITO

INGREDIENTS

- 1 whole-wheat tortilla
- 2 scrambled eggs
- 1/4 cup cooked turkey sausage
- 1/4 cup chopped bell peppers
- 1/4 cup salsa

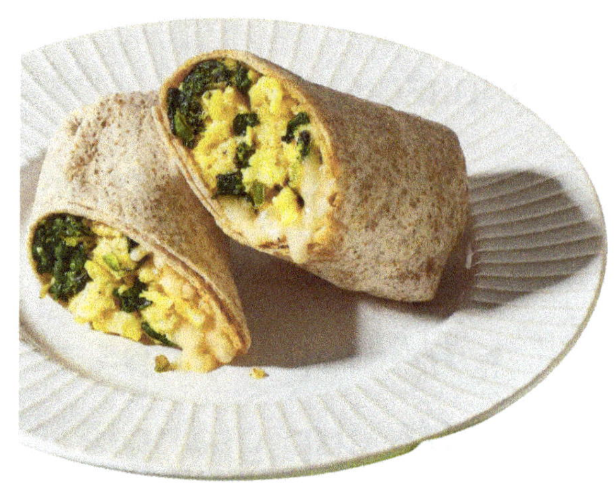

INSTRUCTIONS

1. Warm the tortilla in a skillet over medium heat.
2. Spread scrambled eggs on the tortilla.
3. Top with cooked turkey sausage, chopped bell peppers, and salsa.
4. Roll the tortilla up tightly.
5. Enjoy immediately.

TESTOSTERONE-ENHANCING BREAKFAST SALAD

INGREDIENTS

- **2 cups mixed greens**
- **1/2 cup chopped avocado**
- **1/4 cup cooked chicken or tofu**
- **1/4 cup chopped bell peppers**
- **1 tablespoon olive oil**
- **1 tablespoon balsamic vinegar**

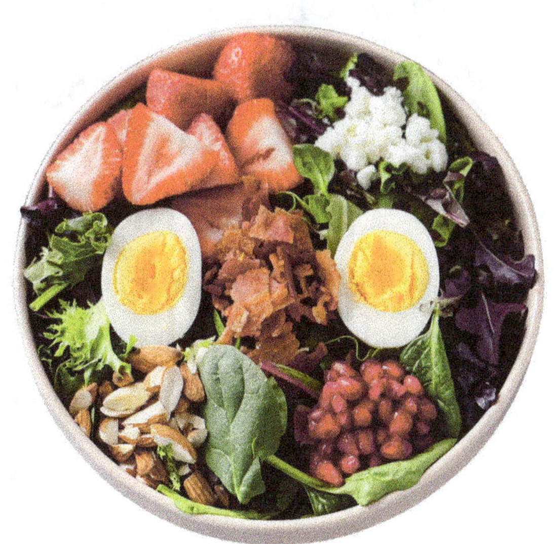

INSTRUCTIONS

Toss together mixed greens, chopped avocado, cooked chicken.

2. Enjoy as you please

TESTOSTERONE-ENHANCING BREAKFAST SANDWICH

INGREDIENTS

- 1 whole-wheat English muffin
- 2 scrambled eggs
- 1 slice cooked turkey sausage
- 1 slice avocado

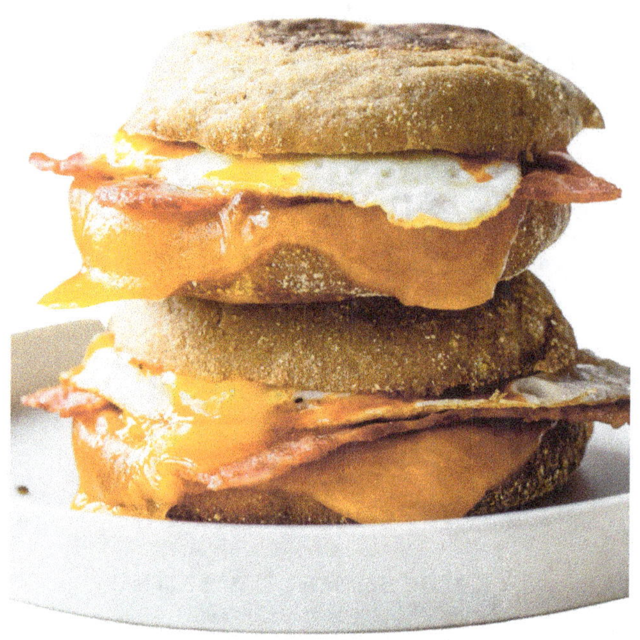

INSTRUCTIONS

1. Toast English muffin to your liking.

2. Spread scrambled eggs on the muffin.

3. Top with cooked turkey sausage and sliced avocado.

4. Enjoy immediately.

TESTOSTERONE-ENHANCING BREAKFAST QUESADILLA

INGREDIENTS

- 1 whole-wheat tortilla
- 1/4 cup shredded cheese
- 2 scrambled eggs
- 1/4 cup chopped bell peppers

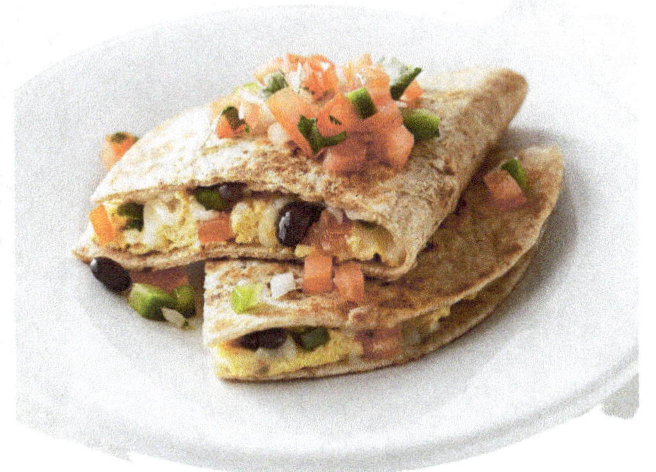

INSTRUCTIONS

1. Spread cheese on one half of the tortilla.

2. Top with scrambled eggs and chopped bell peppers.

3. Fold the tortilla in half.

4. Heat a skillet over medium heat and cook the quesadilla until the cheese is melted and the tortilla is golden brown.

5. Enjoy immediately.

TESTOSTERONE-ENHANCING CHIA SEED PUDDING

INGREDIENTS

- 1/4 cup chia seeds
- 1 cup milk or yogurt
- 1/4 cup berries
- 1 tablespoon honey or maple syrup

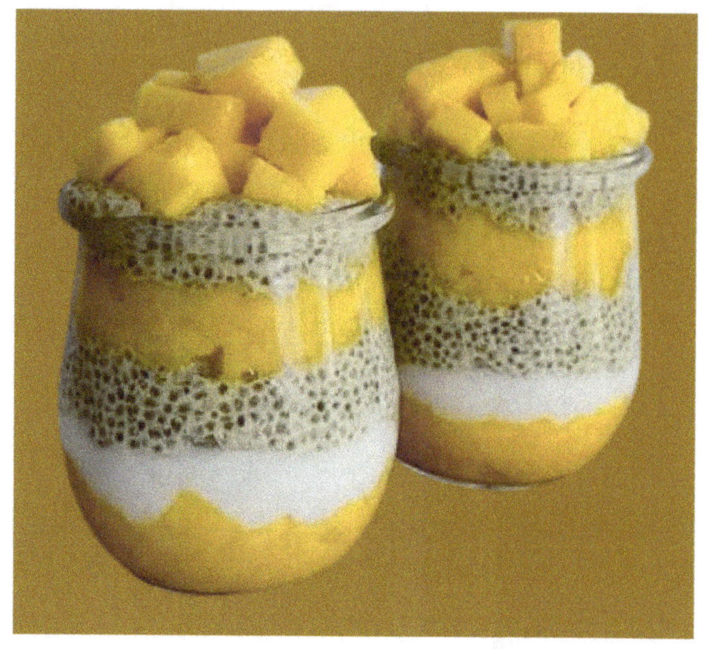

INSTRUCTIONS

1. Combine chia seeds, milk or yogurt, and berries in a jar or container.
2. Stir well and refrigerate overnight.
3. Top with honey or maple syrup and enjoy in the morning.

A Morning Ritual for Hormonal Harmony

Every sunrise is an opportunity to nourish not just our physical bodies but also the core of our well-being. It also holds the promise of a new day and a fresh start. I can attest to the significant influence that adopting healthy breakfast recipes has had on my life, having personally witnessed their transformative effect.

It's simple to forget the importance of breakfast in the daily rush of life. My morning routine for years consisted of getting something quickly in the morning, frequently compromising on nutrition in favor of convenience. I had no idea that I was unintentionally ignoring a vital component of my health: hormonal balance, and specifically the subtle dance that testosterone performs.

After researching the topic of optimal nutrition, I found that breakfast is essential for establishing the hormonal tone of the day, controlling blood sugar levels, and boosting metabolism. My daily routine changed as a result of this realization, and adding nutritious breakfast recipes became a pillar of my wellness path.

It's no longer just a habit for me to eat nutrient-dense meals for breakfast—such as hormone-balancing superfoods, protein-rich smoothies, and hearty whole-grain cereals—but a conscious decision to put my health first. These recipes provide me the energy I need to nourish my body and get through the day without letting me crash in the middle of the morning, which was an all too common occurrence for me.

The biggest shift I observed was in my general attitude and level of concentration. There is no denying the benefits of a well-balanced breakfast for cognitive performance. Having the correct nutrients in my system at the beginning of the day has improved my productivity and creativity by enabling me to approach jobs with efficiency and clarity.

These breakfast recipes have also evolved into a celebration of diversity and taste. I now enjoy the full aromas and textures of healthful products, far from the boring and bland "health foods" I used to associate with breakfast. Breakfast has evolved from a boring old necessity to a gourmet journey, bringing joy and nourishment to every morning.

Probably the most satisfying part is seeing the improvements in my hormonal health. I am more energized, have better-toned muscles, and overall feel better since I started a breakfast regimen designed to augment testosterone production. It feels like my body is saying "thank you" for giving it the fundamental components it requires to survive.

My experience creating healthy breakfast recipes has, in essence, been a revelation—a proof of the significant influence that conscious eating can have on our lives. I'm reminded as I relish every bite of my morning habit that making an investment in a healthy breakfast isn't just about getting a good start to the day; it's also about cultivating a lifestyle that recognizes the remarkable relationship that exists between nutrition and overall wellbeing.
Thus, cheers to breakfasts that satisfy the body and the spirit, to mornings full of energy, and to the never-ending quest to realize the full potential of a happy, healthy existence.

Breakfast Menu

Date :

Sun — Scrambled Egg

Mon

Tue

Wed

Thu

Fri

Sat

Breakfast Menu

Date :

Sun

Mon

Tue

Wed

Thu

Fri

Sat

Breakfast Menu

Date :

Sun

Mon

Tue

Wed

Thu

Fri

Sat

Breakfast Menu

Date :

Sun

Mon

Tue

Wed

Thu

Fri

Sat

Breakfast Menu

Date :

Sun

Mon

Tue

Wed

Thu

Fri

Sat

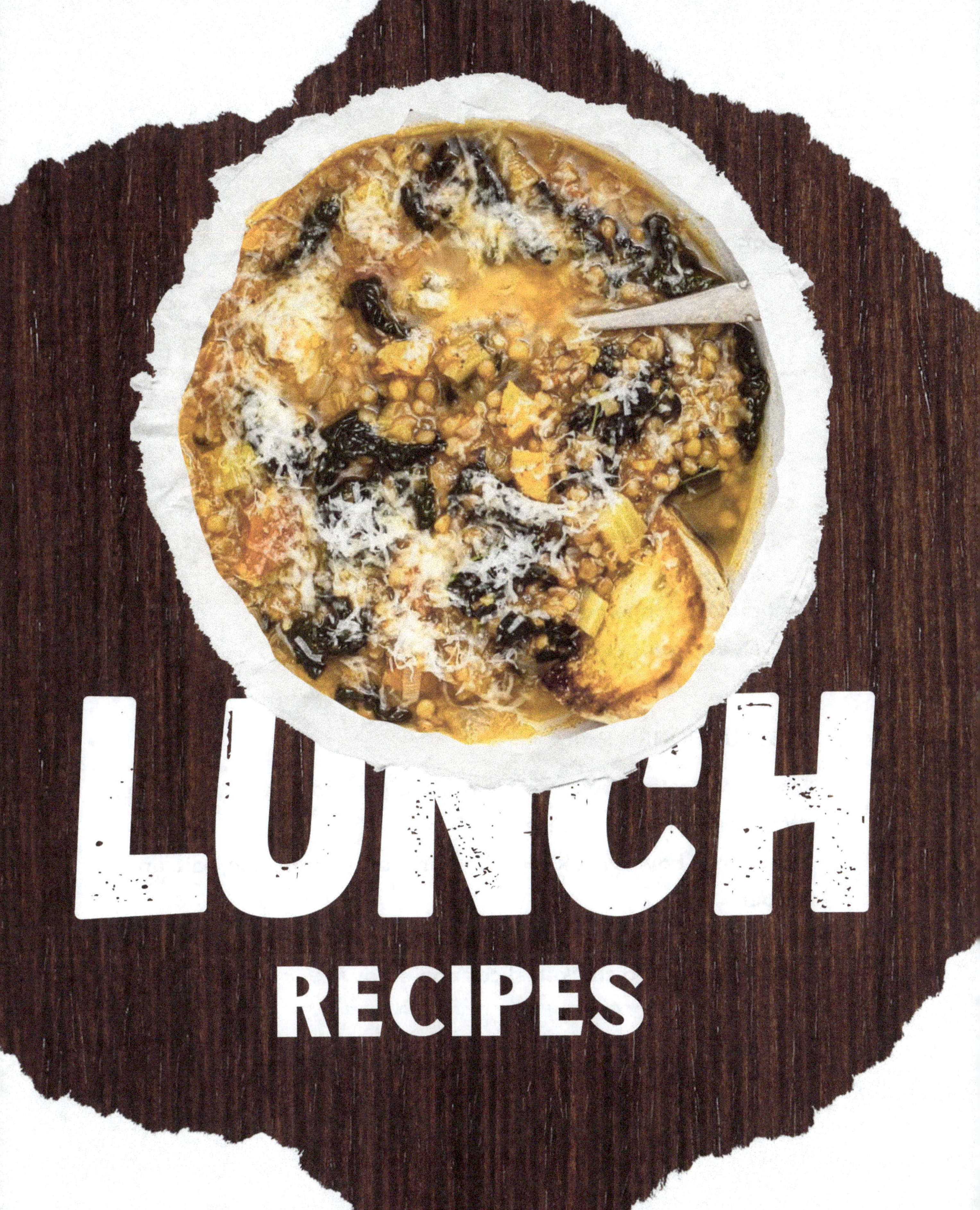

LUNCH
RECIPES

TESTOSTERONE-BOOSTING GRILLED CHICKEN SALAD

INGREDIENTS

- 4 ounces grilled chicken breast, sliced
- 2 cups mixed greens
- 1/2 cup cherry tomatoes, halved
- 1/2 cup cucumber, sliced
- 1/4 cup crumbled feta cheese
- 2 tablespoons extra virgin olive oil
- 1 tablespoon lemon juice
- Salt and pepper to taste

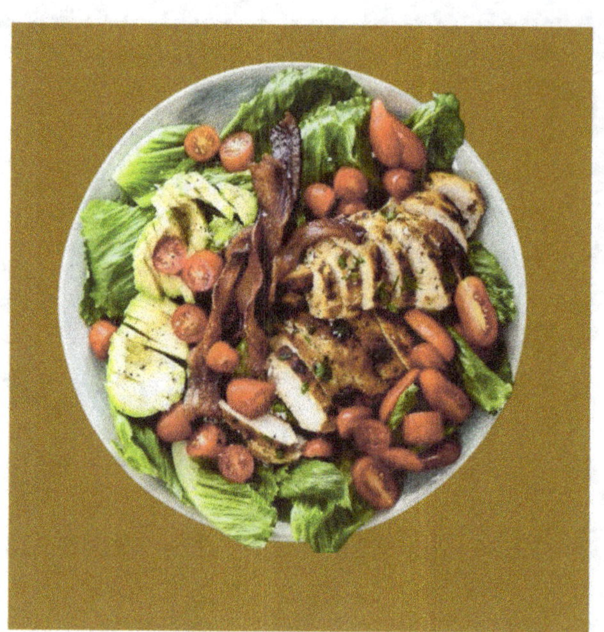

INSTRUCTIONS

1. In a large salad bowl, combine mixed greens, cherry tomatoes, cucumber, and feta cheese.
2. In a small bowl, whisk together olive oil, lemon juice, salt, and pepper.
3. Pour dressing over the salad and toss to coat.
4. Top with grilled chicken slices and enjoy.

TESTOSTERONE-ENHANCING SALMON SALAD WITH AVOCADO AND SPINACH

INGREDIENTS

- **4 ounces cooked salmon, flaked**
- **2 cups baby spinach**
- **1 avocado, diced**
- **1/4 cup red onion, thinly sliced**
- **2 tablespoons olive oil**
- **1 tablespoon lemon juice**
- **Salt and pepper to taste**

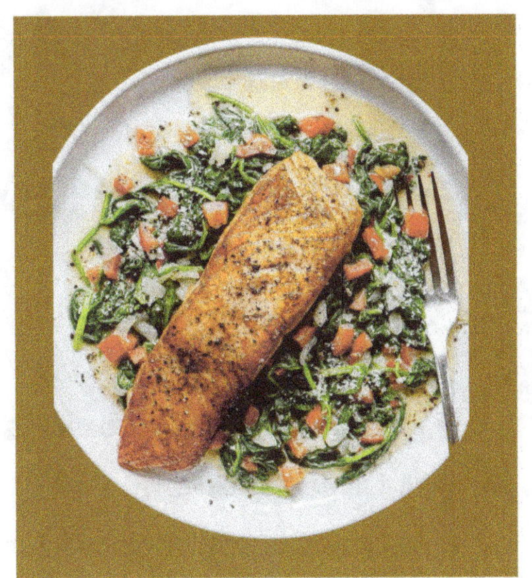

INSTRUCTIONS

1. In a large salad bowl, combine baby spinach, avocado, and red onion.

2. In a small bowl, whisk together olive oil, lemon juice, salt, and pepper.

3. Pour dressing over the salad and toss to coat.

4. Top with flaked salmon and enjoy.

TESTOSTERONE-BOOSTING TURKEY AND QUINOA BOWL

INGREDIENTS

- 1 cup quinoa, cooked
- 4 ounces ground turkey, browned
- 1/2 cup chopped bell peppers
- 1/2 cup chopped onions
- 1 tablespoon olive oil
- 1 teaspoon chili powder
- 1/2 teaspoon cumin
- 1/4 cup salsa
- 1/4 cup avocado, diced

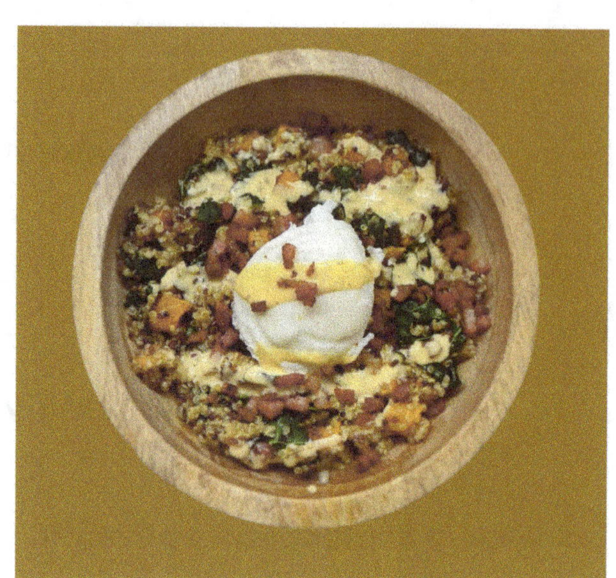

INSTRUCTIONS

1. In a large skillet, heat olive oil over medium heat.

2. Add ground turkey and cook until browned.

3. Add bell peppers and onions and cook until softened.

4. Stir in chili powder and cumin.

5. In a serving bowl, combine cooked quinoa, turkey mixture, salsa, and diced avocado.

6. Enjoy immediately.

TESTOSTERONE-ENHANCING BLACK BEAN BURGERS

INGREDIENTS

- 1 (15-ounce) can black beans, drained and rinsed
- 1 cup cooked brown rice
- 1/4 cup chopped red onion
- 1/4 cup chopped bell pepper
- 1 tablespoon olive oil
- 1 teaspoon cumin
- 1/2 teaspoon chili powder
- Salt and pepper to taste

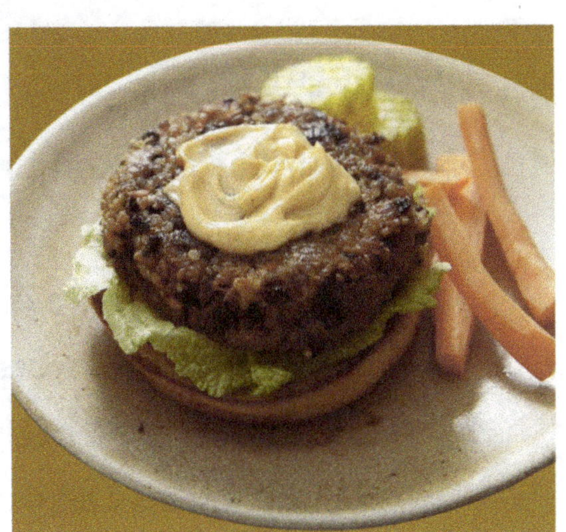

INSTRUCTIONS

1. In a large bowl, mash black beans with a fork until mostly smooth.
2. Add cooked brown rice, red onion, bell pepper, olive oil, cumin, chili powder, salt, and pepper.
3. Mix well until ingredients are evenly distributed.
4. Form the mixture into patties.
5. Heat a skillet over medium heat and cook the burgers until golden brown on both sides.

INGREDIENTS

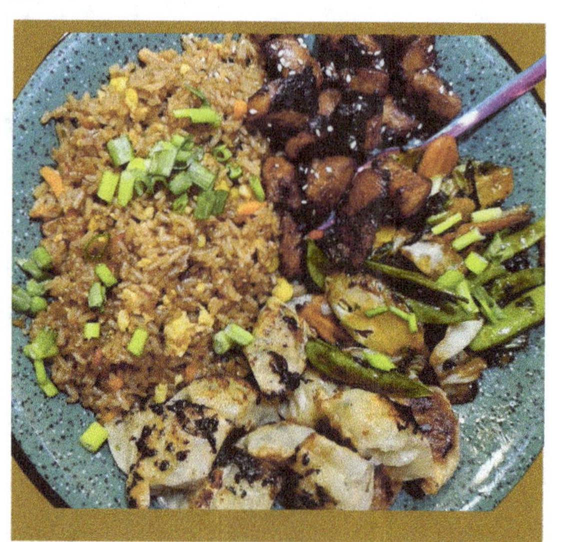

- **4 ounces chicken breast, cut into strips**
- **1 tablespoon olive oil**
- **1 cup broccoli florets**
- **1 cup sliced bell peppers**
- **1/2 cup sliced carrots**
- **1/4 cup soy sauce**
- **1 tablespoon honey**
- **Salt and pepper to taste**

INSTRUCTIONS

1. In a large skillet or wok, heat olive oil over medium-high heat.

2. Add chicken strips and cook until browned on all sides.

3. Add broccoli florets, bell peppers, and carrots.

4. Stir-fry for 3-5 minutes, or until vegetables are tender-crisp.

5. In a small bowl, whisk together soy sauce and honey.

6. Pour the sauce over the stir-fry and cook for 1-2 minutes more, or until the sauce is thickened and heated through.

7. Serve over brown rice or quinoa.

TESTOSTERONE-BOOSTING TUNA SALAD WITH AVOCADO AND SPINACH

INGREDIENTS

- 1 (12-ounce) can tuna, drained
- 1 avocado, mashed
- 1/4 cup chopped red onion
- 1/4 cup chopped celery
- 2 tablespoons olive oil
- 1 tablespoon lemon juice
- Salt and pepper to taste

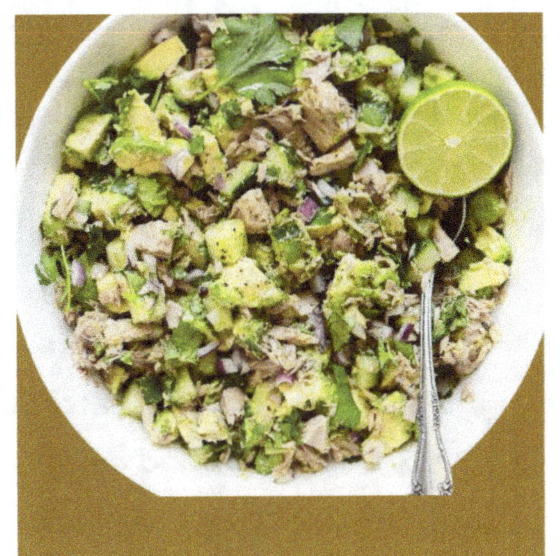

INSTRUCTIONS

1. In a large skillet or wok, heat olive oil over medium-high heat.

2. Add chicken strips and cook until browned on all sides.

3. Add broccoli florets, bell peppers, and carrots.

4. Stir-fry for 3-5 minutes, or until vegetables are tender-crisp.

5. In a small bowl, whisk together soy sauce and honey.

6. Pour the sauce over the stir-fry and cook for 1-2 minutes more, or until the sauce is thickened and heated through.

7. Serve over brown rice or quinoa.

TESTOSTERONE-ENHANCING LENTIL SOUP

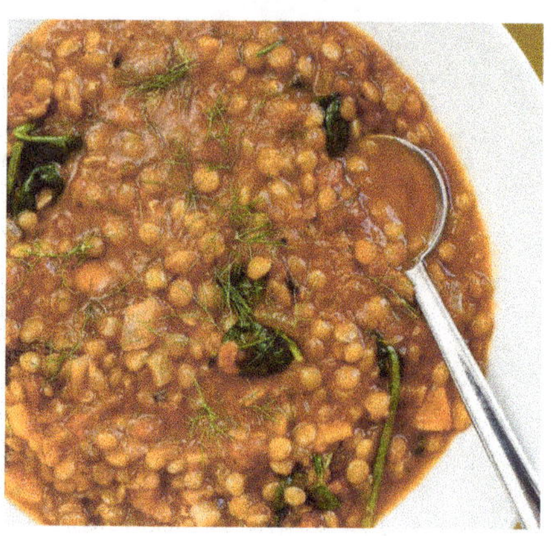

INGREDIENTS

- 1 (15-ounce) can lentils, drained and rinsed
- 1 (14.5-ounce) can diced tomatoes, undrained
- 1 cup vegetable broth
- 1/2 cup chopped carrots
- 1/2 cup chopped celery
- 1/4 cup chopped onion
- 1 tablespoon olive oil
- 1 teaspoon cumin
- 1/2 teaspoon chili powder
- Salt and pepper to taste

INSTRUCTIONS

1. In a large pot, heat olive oil over medium heat.

2. Add carrots, celery, and onion and cook until softened.

3. Stir in cumin and chili powder.

4. Add lentils, diced tomatoes, vegetable broth, salt, and pepper.

5. Bring to a boil, then reduce heat and simmer for 20-30 minutes, or until lentils are tender.

6. Serve with your favorite toppings, such as chopped cilantro, avocado, or sour cream

TESTOSTERONE-BOOSTING SHRIMP SCAMPI

INGREDIENTS
- 1 pound shrimp, peeled and deveined
- 1 tablespoon olive oil
- 4 cloves garlic, minced
- 1/2 cup dry white wine
- 1/2 cup chopped fresh parsley
- 1/4 cup grated Parmesan cheese
- Salt and pepper to taste

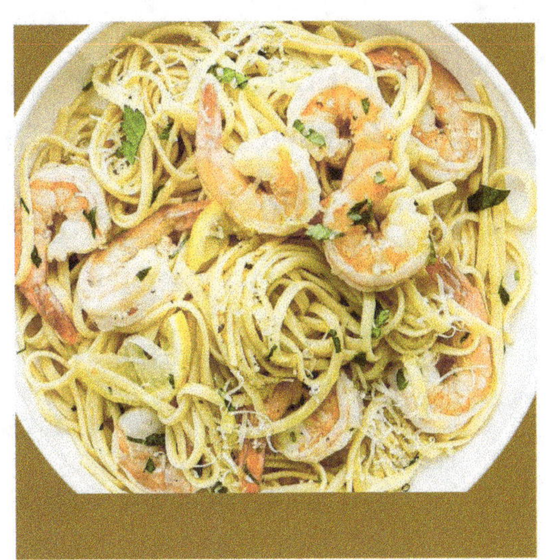

INSTRUCTIONS
1. In a large skillet, heat olive oil over medium heat.

2. Add garlic and cook until fragrant.

3. Add shrimp and cook until pink and curled.

4. Deglaze the pan with white wine, scraping up any browned bits from the bottom of the pan.

5. Stir in parsley, Parmesan cheese, salt, and pepper.

6. Cook for 1-2 minutes more, or until the sauce is thickened and heated through.

7. Serve over pasta or zucchini noodles.

TESTOSTERONE-ENHANCING GRILLED SALMON WITH ROASTED VEGETABLES

INGREDIENTS

- **4 ounces salmon fillet**
- **1 tablespoon olive oil**
- **Salt and pepper to taste**
- **1 cup broccoli florets**
- **1 cup sliced carrots**
- **1/2 cup sliced onions**

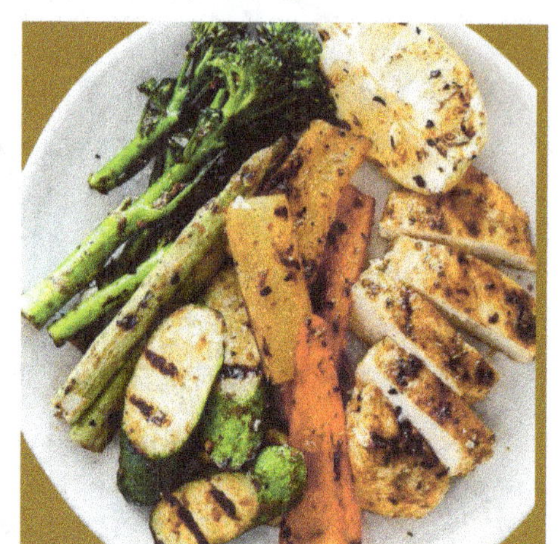

INSTRUCTIONS

1. Preheat oven to 400 degrees F (200 degrees C).

2. Toss broccoli florets, sliced carrots, and sliced onions with olive oil, salt, and pepper.

3. Spread vegetables on a baking sheet and roast for 20-25 minutes, or until tender.

4. While the vegetables are roasting, season the salmon fillet with olive oil, salt, and pepper.

5. Heat a grill pan or grill over medium-high heat.

6. Grill the salmon fillet for 4-5 minutes per side, or until cooked through.

7. Serve the salmon with roasted vegetables.

TESTOSTERONE-ENHANCING CHICKEN AND AVOCADO WRAP

INGREDIENTS

- **4 ounces cooked chicken, shredded**
- **1 whole-wheat tortilla**
- **1/2 avocado, mashed**
- **1/4 cup chopped spinach**
- **1 tablespoon lemon juice**
- **Salt and pepper to taste**

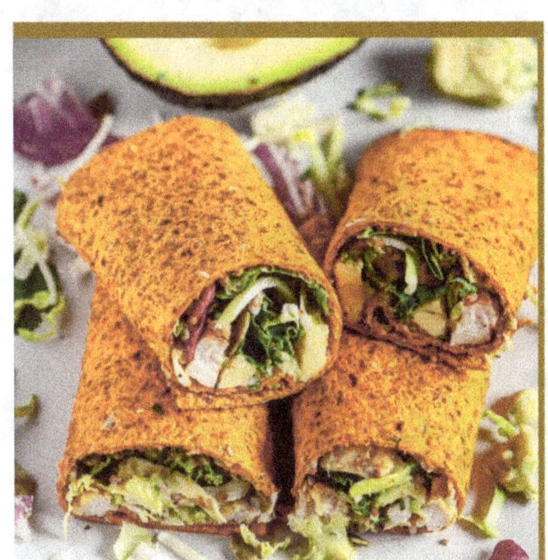

INSTRUCTIONS

1. Spread mashed avocado on the tortilla.

2. Top with shredded chicken, chopped spinach, lemon juice, salt, and pepper.

3. Roll the tortilla up tightly.

4. Cut the wrap in half and enjoy.

LUNCH
Menu

Date :

Sun

Mon

Tue

Wed

Thu

Fri

Sat

LUNCH
Menu

Date :

Sun

Mon

Tue

Wed

Thu

Fri

Sat

LUNCH
Menu

Date :

Sun

Mon

Tue

Wed

Thu

Fri

Sat

LUNCH
Menu

Date :

Sun

Mon

Tue

Wed

Thu

Fri

Sat

LUNCH
Menu

Date :

Sun

Mon

Tue

Wed

Thu

Fri

Sat

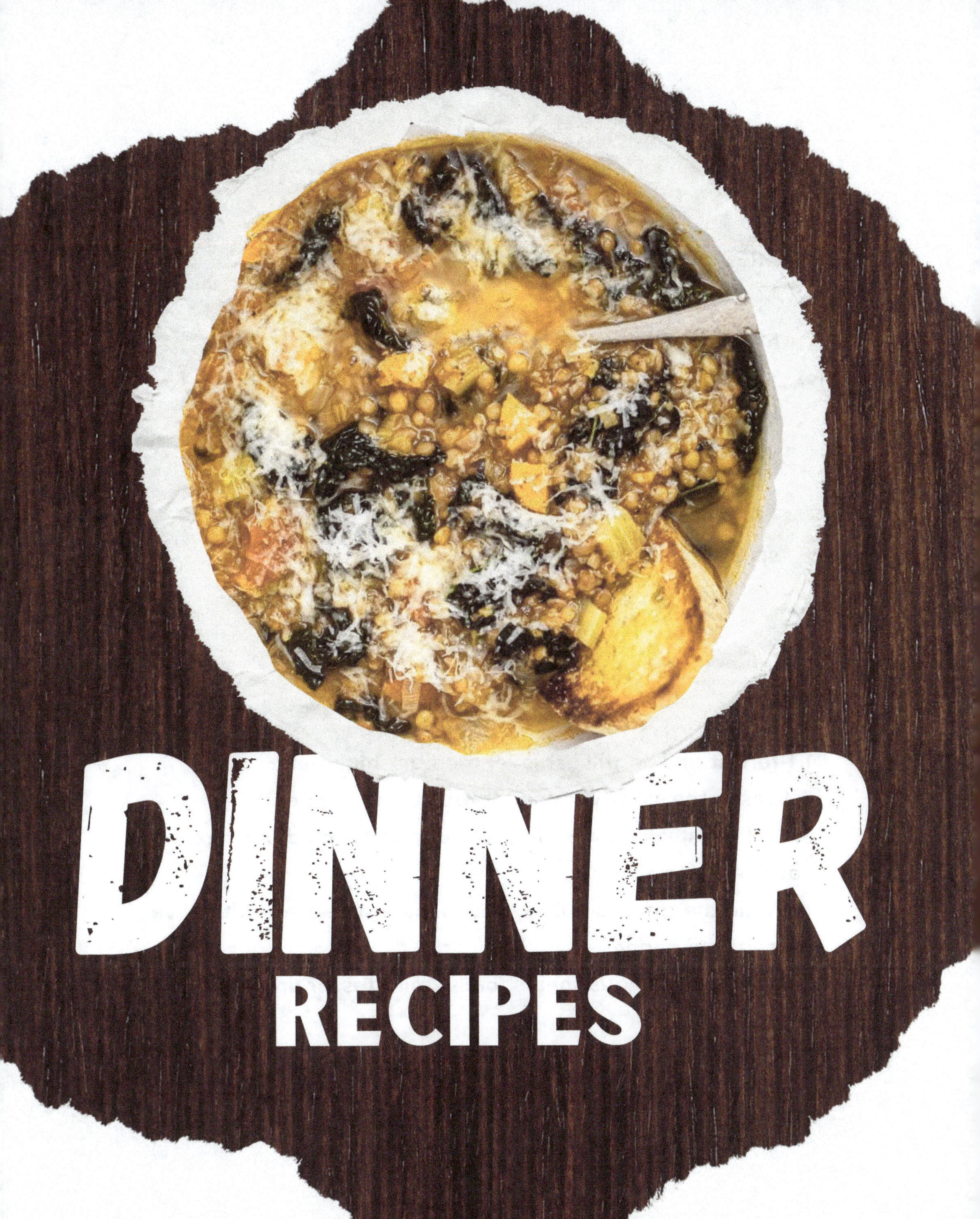

DINNER
RECIPES

TESTOSTERONE-BOOSTING GRILLED STEAK WITH ROASTED ASPARAGUS

INGREDIENTS

- **12 ounces ribeye steak**
- **1 tablespoon olive oil**
- **Salt and pepper to taste**
- **1 pound asparagus spears, trimmed**

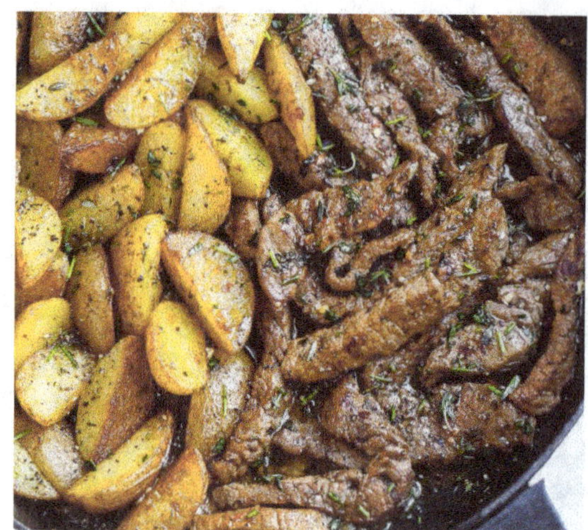

INSTRUCTIONS

1. Preheat grill or grill pan over medium-high heat.
2. Season the steak with olive oil, salt, and pepper.
3. Grill the steak for 4-5 minutes per side for medium-rare, or to your desired doneness.
4. While the steak is grilling, toss asparagus spears with olive oil, salt, and pepper.
5. Grill the asparagus spears for 5-7 minutes, or until tender-crisp.
6. Serve the steak with roasted asparagus.

TESTOSTERONE-ENHANCING SALMON WITH LEMON AND DILL

INGREDIENTS

- 4 ounces salmon fillet
- 1 tablespoon olive oil
- 1 tablespoon lemon juice
- 1 teaspoon dried dill
- Salt and pepper to taste

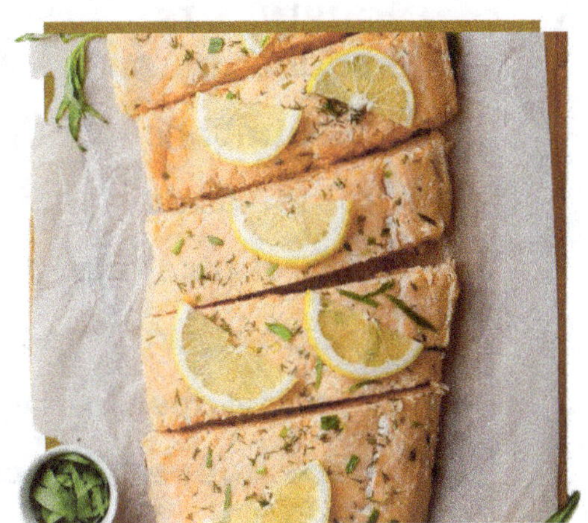

INSTRUCTIONS

1. Preheat oven to 400 degrees F (200 degrees C).
2. Place the salmon fillet on a baking sheet lined with parchment paper.
3. Drizzle the salmon with olive oil and lemon juice.
4. Sprinkle with dried dill, salt, and pepper.
5. Bake for 15-20 minutes, or until cooked through.

TESTOSTERONE-BOOSTING TURKEY CHILI

INGREDIENTS

- 1 pound ground turkey, browned
- 1 (15-ounce) can kidney beans, drained and rinsed
- 1 (14.5-ounce) can diced tomatoes, undrained
- 1 cup chopped onion
- 1 cup chopped bell pepper
- 1 tablespoon olive oil
- 1 tablespoon chili powder
- 1 teaspoon cumin
- 1/2 teaspoon smoked paprika
- Salt and pepper to taste

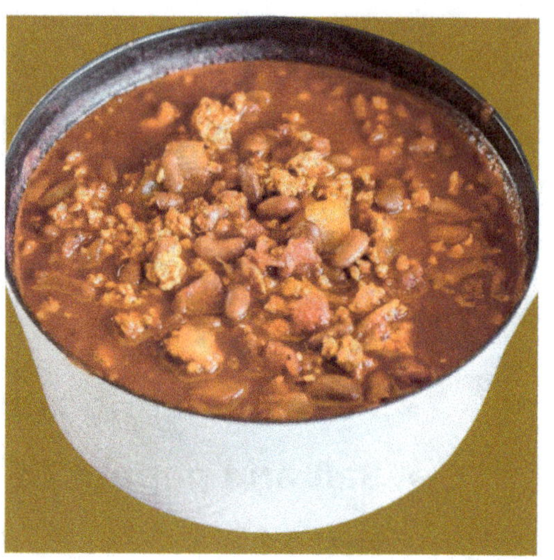

INSTRUCTIONS

1. In a large pot, heat olive oil over medium heat.

2. Add chopped onion and bell pepper and cook until softened.

3. Add ground turkey and cook until browned.

4. Stir in chili powder, cumin, smoked paprika, salt, and pepper.

5. Add kidney beans and diced tomatoes.

6. Bring to a boil, then reduce heat and simmer for 20-30 minutes, or until the chili is thickened.

7. Serve with your favorite toppings, such as avocado, sour cream, or shredded cheese.

TESTOSTERONE-ENHANCING CHICKEN AND SHRIMP STIR-FRY

INGREDIENTS

- 4 ounces chicken breast, cut into strips
- 4 ounces shrimp, peeled and deveined
- 1 tablespoon olive oil
- 1 cup broccoli florets
- 1 cup sliced bell peppers
- 1/2 cup chopped carrots
- 1/4 cup soy sauce
- 1 tablespoon honey
- Salt and pepper to taste

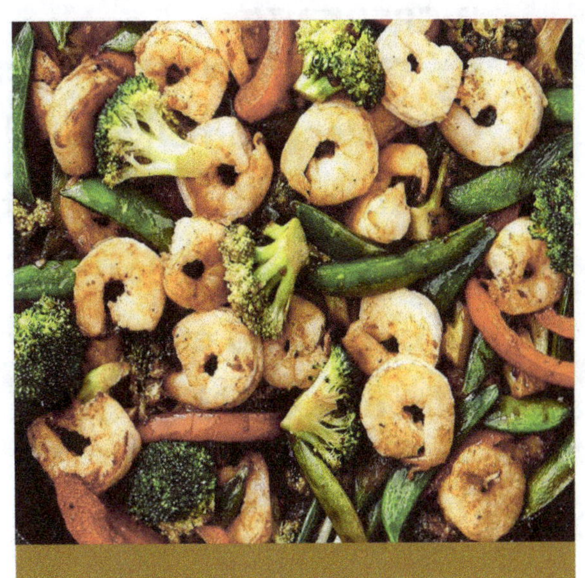

INSTRUCTIONS

1. In a large skillet or wok, heat olive oil over medium-high heat.

2. Add chicken strips and shrimp and cook until browned and cooked through.

3. Add broccoli florets, bell peppers, and carrots.

4. Stir-fry for 3-5 minutes, or until vegetables are tender-crisp.

5. In a small bowl, whisk together soy sauce and honey.

6. Pour the sauce over the stir-fry and cook for 1-2 minutes more, or until the sauce is thickened and heated through.

7. Serve over brown rice or quinoa.

TESTOSTERONE-ENHANCING GRILLED CHICKEN BREAST WITH ROASTED VEGETABLES

INGREDIENTS

- **4 ounces chicken breast**
- **1 tablespoon olive oil**
- **Salt and pepper to taste**
- **1 cup broccoli florets**
- **1 cup sliced carrots**
- **1/2 cup sliced onions**

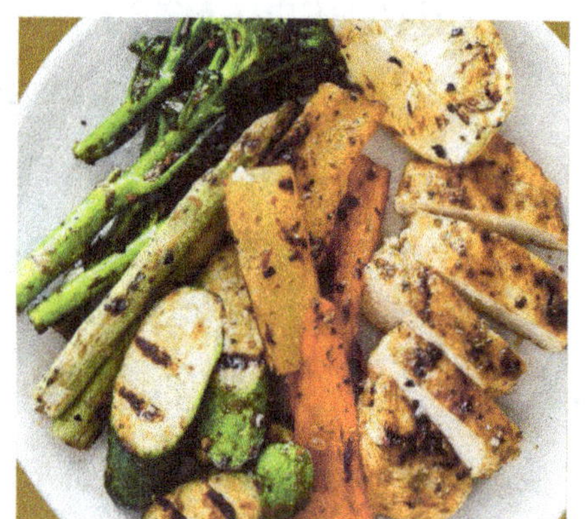

INSTRUCTIONS

1. **Preheat the oven to 400 degrees Fahrenheit.**
2. **In a large bowl, combine the chicken breasts, olive oil, salt, pepper, garlic powder, onion powder, paprika, and cayenne pepper (if using). Toss to coat.**
3. **Place the chicken breasts on a baking sheet and bake for 15-20 minutes, or until cooked through.**
4. **While the chicken is baking, toss the broccoli, Brussels sprouts, sweet potato, and red onion with the olive oil, salt, and pepper in a large bowl.**
5. **Spread the vegetables on a baking sheet and roast for 20-25 minutes, or until tender.**
6. **To serve, slice the chicken breasts and serve with the roasted vegetables.**

TESTOSTERONE-ENHANCING BAKED COD WITH LEMON AND HERBS

INGREDIENTS

- 4 ounces cod fillet
- 1 tablespoon olive oil
- 1 lemon, thinly sliced
- 1 teaspoon dried thyme
- Salt and pepper to taste

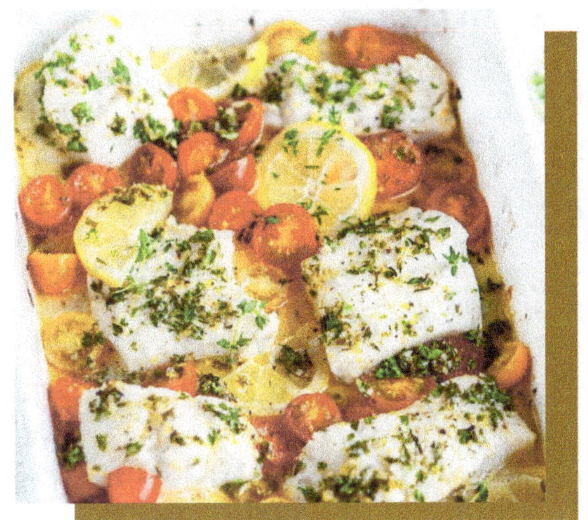

INSTRUCTIONS

1. Preheat oven to 400 degrees F (200 degrees C).

2. Place the cod fillet on a baking sheet lined with parchment paper.

3. Drizzle the cod with olive oil.

4. Top with lemon slices, dried thyme, salt, and pepper.

5. Bake for 15-20 minutes, or until cooked through

TESTOSTERONE-ENHANCING SHRIMP SCAMPI WITH ZUCCHINI NOODLES

INGREDIENTS

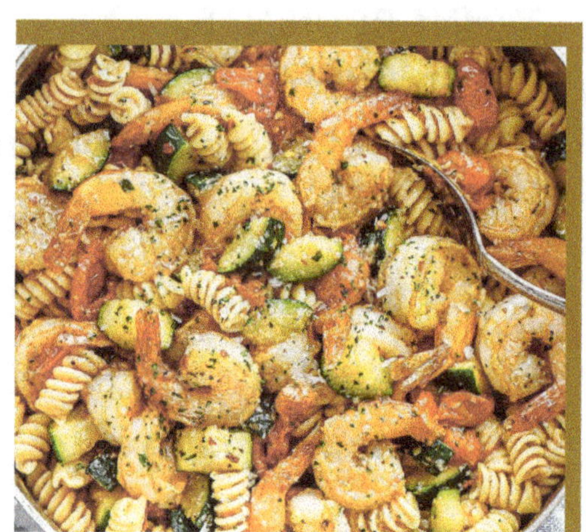

- 1 pound shrimp, peeled and deveined
- 1 tablespoon olive oil
- 4 cloves garlic, minced
- 1/2 cup dry white wine
- 1/2 cup chopped fresh parsley
- 1/4 cup grated Parmesan cheese
- Salt and pepper to taste
- 2 medium zucchini, spiralized into noodles

INSTRUCTIONS

1. In a large skillet, heat olive oil over medium heat.
2. Add garlic and cook until fragrant.
3. Add shrimp and cook until pink and curled.
4. Deglaze the pan with white wine, scraping up any browned bits from the bottom of the pan.
5. Stir in parsley, Parmesan cheese, salt, and pepper.
6. Add zucchini noodles and cook for 1-2 minutes, or until heated through.
7. Serve immediately.

TESTOSTERONE-ENHANCING CHICKEN AND SWEET POTATO SKILLET

INGREDIENTS

- **4 ounces chicken breast, cut into bite-sized pieces**
- **1 tablespoon olive oil**
- **1 medium sweet potato, peeled and diced**
- **1 red bell pepper, diced**
- **1 onion, diced**
- **1 tablespoon chili powder**
- **1 teaspoon cumin**
- **Salt and pepper to taste**

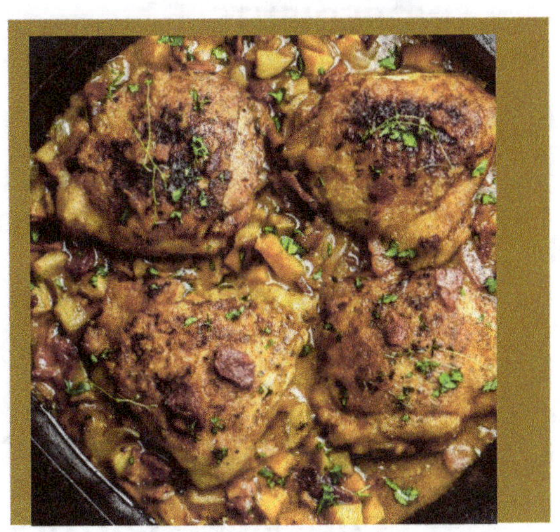

INSTRUCTIONS

1. In a large skillet, heat olive oil over medium heat.
2. Add chicken pieces and cook until browned.
3. Add sweet potato, bell pepper, and onion.
4. Cook until vegetables are tender-crisp.
5. Stir in chili powder, cumin, salt, and pepper.
6. Cook for 1-2 minutes more, or until the spices are fragrant.
7. Serve with your favorite toppings, such as avocado, sour cream, or shredded cheese.

TESTOSTERONE-ENHANCING TUNA SALAD STUFFED AVOCADOS

INGREDIENTS

- **4 ounces salmon fillet**
- **1 tablespoon olive oil**
- **Salt and pepper to taste**
- **1 cup broccoli florets**
- **1 cup sliced carrots**
- **1/2 cup sliced onions**

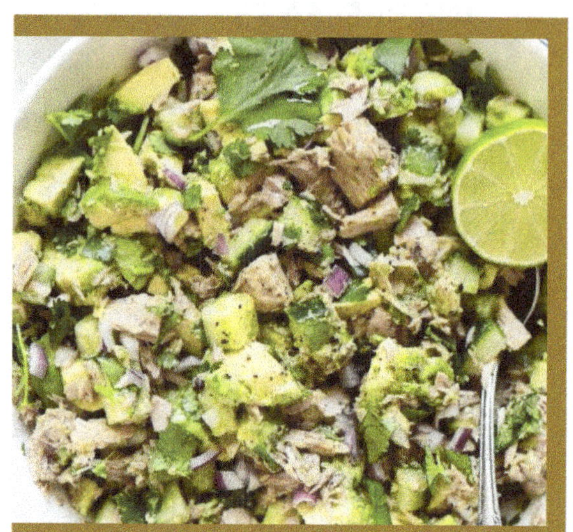

INSTRUCTIONS

1. Preheat oven to 400 degrees F (200 degrees C).
2. Toss broccoli florets, sliced carrots, and sliced onions with olive oil, salt, and pepper.
3. Spread vegetables on a baking sheet and roast for 20-25 minutes, or until tender.
4. While the vegetables are roasting, season the salmon fillet with olive oil, salt, and pepper.
5. Heat a grill pan or grill over medium-high heat.
6. Grill the salmon fillet for 4-5 minutes per side, or until cooked through.
7. Serve the salmon with roasted vegetables.

TESTOSTERONE-ENHANCING GRILLED CHICKEN CAESAR SALAD

INGREDIENTS

- **4 ounces chicken breast, grilled and sliced**
- **2 cups romaine lettuce**
- **1/2 cup grated Parmesan cheese**
- **1/4 cup croutons**
- **Caesar salad dressing**

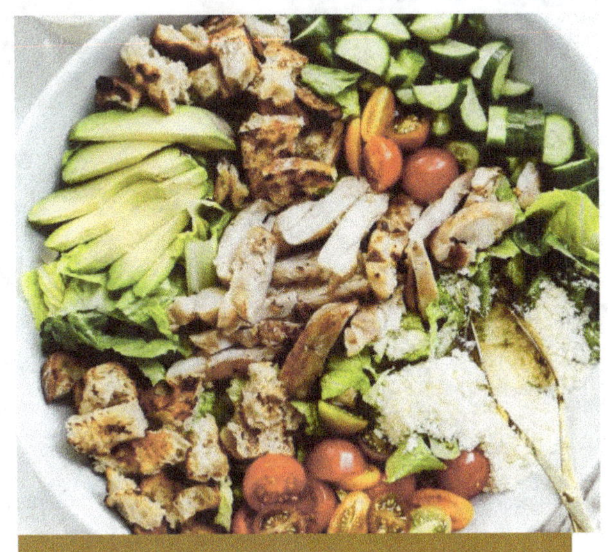

INSTRUCTIONS

1. In a large salad bowl, combine romaine lettuce, Parmesan cheese, and croutons.

2. Add grilled chicken slices.

3. Drizzle with Caesar salad dressing and toss to coat.

4. Enjoy immediately

DINNER
Menu

Date :

Sun

Mon

Tue

Wed

Thu

Fri

Sat

DINNER
Menu

Date :

Sun

Mon

Tue

Wed

Thu

Fri

Sat

DINNER Menu

Date :

Sun

Mon

Tue

Wed

Thu

Fri

Sat

DINNER Menu

Date :

Sun

Mon

Tue

Wed

Thu

Fri

Sat

DINNER
Menu

Date :

Sun

Mon

Tue

Wed

Thu

Fri

Sat

Testosterone-Boosting Snacks and Drinks

As a fitness enthusiast and avid health advocate, I've always been fascinated by the intricate relationship between nutrition, exercise, and hormone balance. Testosterone, the primary male sex hormone, plays a crucial role in muscle growth, energy levels, and overall well-being. While lifestyle factors such as sleep and stress management are essential for optimizing testosterone production, diet also plays a significant role.

Here, I've compiled a list of testosterone-boosting snacks and drinks that can easily be incorporated into a healthy and balanced lifestyle:

Testosterone-Boosting Snack

Nuts and Seeds: Almonds, walnuts, Brazil nuts, sunflower seeds, and pumpkin seeds are all excellent sources of zinc, magnesium, and vitamin E, nutrients that support testosterone production.

Eggs: Eggs are a nutrient-rich food that provides protein, zinc, and vitamin D, all of which contribute to healthy testosterone levels.

Greek Yogurt: Greek yogurt is a protein-packed snack that also contains zinc and magnesium.

Avocado: Avocados are a rich source of healthy fats, fiber, and vitamin D, all of which can support testosterone production.

Berries: Berries, such as blueberries, strawberries, and raspberries, are high in antioxidants and anti-inflammatory compounds that may help boost testosterone levels.

Dark Chocolate: Dark chocolate, with a cocoa content of 70% or higher, contains antioxidants and flavonoids that may help promote healthy testosterone levels.

Testosterone-Boosting Drinks

Water: Staying hydrated is crucial for overall health and may also support testosterone production.

Green Tea: Green tea is rich in catechins, antioxidants that may help boost testosterone levels.

Coffee: Coffee, in moderate amounts, may help increase testosterone levels.

Pomegranate Juice: Pomegranate juice contains antioxidants and anti-inflammatory compounds that may help enhance testosterone production.

Vegetable Juices: Vegetable juices, particularly those containing leafy green vegetables, can provide a concentrated dose of nutrients that support testosterone production.

Consistency is key when it comes to reaping the benefits of testosterone-boosting foods and drinks. By incorporating these nutrient-rich options into your daily routine, you can support optimal hormone balance, enhance your overall health, and experience a surge of energy to power your day.

Overcoming Nutrition Challenges

It's a pleasant path to optimize testosterone through nutrition, but like with any worthy undertaking, there are obstacles along the way. Having personally adopted the Testosterone Advantage lifestyle, I am aware of the potential obstacles and how crucial it is to get past them in order to experience long-term success. We'll explore some of the typical nutrition obstacles encountered on this trip in this chapter, and we'll offer our own perspectives and solutions.

1. Time Restraints: The Never-ending Battle
Lack of time is one of the biggest obstacles to sticking to a diet that is testosterone-friendly. Finding the time to make healthful meals might seem like a Herculean challenge in a world that appears to move at an ever-accelerating pace.

From a personal standpoint, I discovered that making food preparation a priority in my routine was unavoidable after witnessing the daily chaos. I started setting out Sunday evenings to chop veggies, marinate proteins, and arrange portioned containers for the coming week. This easy process guaranteed that I always had a testosterone-optimized meal ready to go, and it also saved me time during hectic workdays.

2. Travel Temptations: Maintaining Your Testosterone Level While Traveling
It can seem logistically difficult to maintain a healthy diet for people who are constantly on the go, whether for work or play. For individuals looking for hormone-friendly meals, fast food restaurants and airport terminals frequently provide few options.

From a personal standpoint, I can say that I have experienced the lure of airport convenience stores and fast-food drive-thrus. I took the initiative in these circumstances and packed my own snacks. Protein bars, nuts, and seeds became my go-to snacks when traveling because they were easy to carry and packed with testosterone compared to the typical fare. Being organized in advance becomes essential to driving on course.

3. Social Environments: Manoeuvring Hormone-Inhibiting Menus
While dining out is a beloved social pastime, maintaining a testosterone-friendly diet can be difficult when doing so. Many restaurant menus provide a wide range of options, not all of them are in line with our dietary objectives.

Personal Viewpoint: I've learnt to see a restaurant's menu as a creative opportunity rather than something that limits me. I discovered that I could still have a beautiful meal and adhere to my testosterone-boosting beliefs by gently seeking alterations from many chefs, who are more than happy to make accommodations for dietary preferences. It all comes down to striking a balance between living in the present and taking care of your health.

4. desires: The War of the Sweet Tooth Sweet desires can be strong rivals when it comes to sticking to a diet that maximizes testosterone in the body. Even the most self-controlling people can be put to the test by the appeal of sweets and desserts.

Personal View: Rather than completely giving in to my sweet tooth, I accepted the task of finding dessert options that would appeal to men more than women. Recipes using natural sweeteners, such as honey or maple syrup, met my need for sweetness without sacrificing any of my dietary objectives. It all comes down to making decisions that support your health and happiness.

5. Financial Restraints: Fueling Your Hormones on a Budget
Healthy eating is frequently more expensive, and for many people, this financial barrier is a major obstacle.

Personal Viewpoint: Having lived through financial hardships, I discovered that, by carefully considering my options and giving some foods priority over others, I could optimize my nutritious intake without going over budget. Purchasing in large quantities, choosing seasonal food, and investigating nearby marketplaces were a few of the tactics I employed to fuel my body without breaking the bank.

6. Maintaining Motivation: A Long-Term View
Sustaining motivation over the long term may be the journey's most persistent problem. The initial zeal for testosterone-optimized nutrition may fade and be eclipsed by the comfort of old habits, as is the case with any lifestyle change.

From a personal standpoint, I battled this difficulty by remembering my long-term objectives. I thought back to the good things that had happened to me: more energy, a happier mood, and an overall sense of well-being. Establishing a connection with the wider advantages that go beyond testosterone optimization supplied the internal drive required to maintain this way of life. Sharing the journey with like-minded people also created a network of accountability and support, whether through local support groups or online forums.

Conquering nutrition obstacles on the way to a Testosterone Advantage lifestyle necessitates a combination of doable tactics and a strong mentality. Through accepting these obstacles as chances for development and education and exchanging experiences in a friendly group, we can manage the intricacies of everyday existence while adhering to our dedication to hormonal well-being. Recall that this is a lifetime investment in your health, not just a diet.

Sustaining the Testosterone Advantage: Long-Term Strategies

The emphasis now is on maintaining the Testosterone Advantage over the long haul as we set out on the last part of our testosterone-boosting adventure. After overcoming obstacles and seeing the transformational potential of diet, this chapter delves into the author's observations and understandings of developing long-lasting plans for hormonal health that last a lifetime.

1. Building Sustainable Habits: A Way of Life, Not Just a Trend
It takes a marathon to optimize testosterone levels rather than a sprint. From a personal standpoint, I've learned that long-lasting transformation is built on sustainable behaviors. It's about making testosterone-boosting concepts a part of your everyday routine rather than following an arbitrary program.

From a personal standpoint, I tried with a variety of nutritional regimens early on in my journey, some more radical than others. I found that the adjustments that I could just as easily incorporate into my daily routine were the most long-lasting. Rather than adhering to an inflexible schedule, I concentrated on making tiny, doable changes that I could easily sustain over time. This mental change made the goal of hormonal health a lifetime commitment rather than a passing fancy.

2. Intentional Dining: The Skill of Creating a Bond with Food
Eating has become a rushed activity in our fast-paced culture, frequently detachable from the sensory experience of appreciating each bite. On the other side, mindful eating entails developing an appreciation and awareness for the food we eat.

From a personal standpoint, I feel that adopting mindful eating techniques has changed my life. Savoring each meal's flavors, textures, and scents not only improves the eating experience but also helps people develop a stronger bond with the food's nutritional value. My commitment to long-term well-being was strengthened by the increased satisfaction I experienced from testosterone-boosting meals when I was able to fully appreciate the nutrients on a sensory level.

3. Adjusting to Changing Requirements: The Rhythms of Life
Both life and our nutritional demands are dynamic. Maintaining the Testosterone Advantage requires constant adjustment to meet our body' changing needs and way of life.

From a personal standpoint, I have come to understand how crucial it is to continue paying attention to the cues that my body gives me. My nutritional strategy had to be adjusted due to variations in activity levels, lifestyle changes, and hormonal shifts. I was able to keep the Testosterone Advantage throughout my life by accepting change and being willing to adjust my eating patterns.

4. Ongoing Education: Providing Knowledge to Empower
A powerful weapon in the pursuit of long-term testosterone optimization is knowledge. Making educated decisions is facilitated by staying up to date on the most recent findings, dietary recommendations, and developments in the field of hormonal health.

From a personal standpoint, I've discovered that the more I learn about the science underlying nutrition and testosterone, the better-equipped I am to make decisions that support my long-term objectives. Staying up to date on new recipes and culinary techniques, or comprehending the effects of particular nutrients, ongoing education has become a crucial aspect of my journey. This information not only reaffirms my dedication but also adds new dimensions of delight to my continuing investigation into testosterone-promoting eating.

5. Creating a Helping Community: The Power of Numbers
Entering the Testosterone Advantage program is a team effort. Creating and maintaining a community of support can offer the shared experiences, accountability, and encouragement needed for long-term success.

Personal Viewpoint: I've found inspiration and motivation in connecting with people who have similar aims to mine. The feeling of community has been a pillar of my continued dedication, whether we are talking about difficulties, exchanging recipes, or commemorating successes. Resilience and perseverance can be fostered by joining friends and family in the trip, participating in online forums, or even just asking for help.

6. Examining Developments: Honoring the Trip
Recognizing and appreciating personal development is essential to long-term testosterone optimization. Examining advancements not only fosters a feeling of success but also highlights the Testosterone Advantage's importance as a life-changing experience.

From a personal standpoint, pausing to consider how far I've come has been crucial to keeping up my dedication. Not only should physical changes be noted, but also good changes in energy, mood, and general well-being. Seeing the event as a whole has given me newfound determination to keep taking care of my hormonal balance.

To sum up, maintaining the Testosterone Advantage entails a continuous process that includes developing thoughtful routines, being flexible, learning new things, forming communities, and enjoying the trip. As we adopt these long-term tactics, let's keep in mind that maintaining hormonal health is a journey that is well worth the work rather than a destination. I hope that the Testosterone Advantage lifestyle will provide you with longevity, strength, and vigor.